Pegan Diet

Exquisite Culinary Preparations, Comprehensive Dietary
Programs, And Beneficial Insights For Novices To
Attain Optimal Well-being And Long-term Weight
Management

(The Cookbook Of Paleo & Vegan Diets)

Steven Levasseur

TABLE OF CONTENT

What Is The Pegan Diet?

Combining elements of the paleo and vegetarian diets, the Pegan diet diverges significantly from conventional dietary approaches.

Initially, it seems to be the case that the Paleo diet is being followed, as it involves the consumption of high-quality meats, eggs, and animal fats. Hence, the vegetarian diet, which intentionally avoids any derivatives stemming from animals, is in direct opposition. The term "pegan" was coined by Dr. Mark Hyman in a blog post on his website that was published on November 7, 2014. The director of the Cleveland Clinic Center for Functional Medicine affirmed that his decision to integrate elements of the paleo and vegetarian diets stemmed from scientific evidence indicating that both approaches possess attributes conducive to promoting overall well-being. Both proponents of the paleo and vegetarian diets are recognized for promoting sustainable weight loss, reducing cholesterol levels, and reversing the development of diabetes. However, considering the significant disparities between these two methodologies, which one is the appropriate alternative? Hyman advises that you embody both characteristics. According to Hyman's distinctive pegan blog post, he expressed, "I have made the conscious decision to embrace the pegan or paleo-vegetarian lifestyle, not only for myself but also as a recommendation for a significant portion of my patients." It is important to bear in mind that individuals were able to tailor the approach based on their medical condition, preferences, and requirements."

The Pegan diet merges the principles of the Paleo diet and vegetarian diet, primarily based on the premise that consuming nutrient-dense, whole foods is associated with a reduction in blood sugar levels, inflammation, and weight, and has been proven to sustain a healthy weight in the long run. Despite its designation, the dietary regimen is noteworthy due to its unique set of guidelines for individuals adhering to a Pegan lifestyle. It is not nearly as restrictive as the paleo or vegetarian diet. The primary advantages that contribute to the overall improvement of individuals' well-being, for those adhering to a Pegan diet, lie in their consumption of novel foods cultivated at ground level. However, it should be noted that this diet also allows for the consumption of limited amounts of meat, fish, poultry, nuts, seeds, and vegetables. Furthermore, small amounts of prepared food options, oils, grains, and sugars continue to be permissible.

Guidelines pertaining to the Pegan Diet

When informed individuals are made aware that this dietary plan encompasses elements of both the paleolithic and vegetarian regimens, they typically anticipate a merger of the shared aspects of these two diets in practical terms. Nevertheless, the limited overlap in food options between the two primarily consists of organic produce, vegetables, nuts, and seeds, comprising a diet that is undoubtedly characterized by a desire for well-being and health. Taking into account all factors, Hyman asserts that the fundamental focus between the paleo diet and maintaining a healthy vegetarian lifestyle lies in the emphasis on "authentic, unprocessed, fresh food that is sustainably sourced."

The principles endorsed by both dietary regimens, as outlined by Hyman in his original pegan article, are:

A plethora of vegetables and all-natural products.

Substantially reducing glycemic load (significantly lessening the intake of sugar, flour, and refined starches)

Locally sourced, fresh, and cultivated produce that adheres to organic principles, devoid of pesticides, antibiotics, hormones, and genetically modified organisms (GMOs).

Sufficient protein consumption Adequate protein consumption Satisfactory protein intake Sustaining protein intake Sufficient protein ingestion.

Food products devoid of synthetic ingredients, additives, artificial colors, preservatives, monosodium glutamate (MSG), and artificial sweeteners.

Increased consumption of high-quality omega-3 fatty acids.

When considering the rationale behind combining paleo principles with vegetarianism, it is imperative to focus on the procurement of ethically sourced animal products, such as those derived from animals that are wild-caught, free-range, and pasture-fed. Fish should possess low levels of mercury and toxic substances, just as sardines, herring, mackerel, and anchovies do. It is imperative to maintain a considerable distance from fish such as swordfish and Chilean ocean bass, as their mercury levels are significantly elevated. While there may be general agreement between paleo and vegetarian eaters regarding the previous suggestions, certain aspects of the pegan diet may present challenges or reservations for individuals from both dietary backgrounds. In such instances, Hyman substantiates his recommendations through the use of scholarly research.

A Primer On The Pegan Diet

Upon a careful examination of the intricacies inherent in the principles of both the Paleo and Vegan diets, one may find oneself inquisitive as to the plausibility of harmonizing these seemingly disparate approaches in order to forge an innovative dietary regimen. Indeed, the former involves menus that predominantly feature meat, whereas the latter centers around recipes that predominantly emphasize plant-based ingredients. However, this phenomenon can be regarded as a remarkable achievement, as exemplified by the Pegan diet. One must simply assimilate the most advantageous components from each program and tailor them to suit one's specific requirements. It should be observed that Peganism does not purport to possess stringent dietary regulations or schemes. You are encouraged to partake in the consumption of the culinary delights that have always brought you pleasure, albeit in measured and prudent quantities. It is recognized that engaging in physical activity is essential for the proper digestion of food, regardless of the specific nutritional approach one adopts.

Which food items are recommended to be included in a Pegan diet?

We highly recommend ensuring an ample supply of fresh fruits and vegetables. In addition to these options, one may consider including a variety of nuts and seeds, legumes, flaxseed oil, olive oil, walnut oil, as well as coconut and avocado. Eggs can contribute positively to one's health, assuming they are incorporated into one's dietary choices. Individuals who possess a preference for food derived from animals may consider selecting seafood, diverse varieties of fish, and meat procured from animals fed on a grass-based diet. In essence, it is advisable to fully capitalize on the provisions of the natural world, with the objective of acquiring lean sources of protein, nutritious and superior fats, pivotal vitamins and minerals, and judicious carbohydrates. It is of utmost importance to maintain your glycemic load within the parameters of normalcy. In order to achieve this objective, it is advisable to refrain from consuming processed foods that contain excessive amounts of chemical preservatives, sugar, and salt. Indeed, followers of the

Pegan diet ought to endeavor to adhere to domestically sourced or organically grown foods to the greatest extent feasible. Regardless of the circumstances, it is imperative to ensure that approximately 75% of your dietary regimen centers around plant-based offerings, with the remaining portion dedicated to animal-derived options. Exercise moderation when imposing strict limitations upon your taste buds.

For instance, how would an average daily menu be structured?

One way to rephrase this sentence in a more formal tone could be: "To commence your day, you may opt for a medley of berries, assorted nuts, almond butter, almond milk, coconut butter, and a selection of seeds, which can be ingeniously combined to concoct an indulgent protein smoothie." For the midday meal, you can primarily emphasize a salad comprised of avocado, assorted seeds, sardines, or seafood sourced from the wild. The evening meal could include a blend of vegetarian and non-vegetarian dishes. Ensure that the dining table is furnished with a selection of two or three vegetable dishes, complemented by ethically sourced wild-caught fish or locally raised, organic lamb/chicken. Please be advised that the provided content is solely meant to serve as an illustration. You are encouraged to generate a multitude of original adaptations.

What dietary restrictions does the Pegan diet entail?

It is anticipated that you will curtail your consumption of salt, processed foods, processed sugar, the majority of legumes, cereal grains, refined vegetable oils, and dairy products to the greatest extent feasible. Indeed, you may opt to altogether avoid them should you so choose.

Stewed Collard Greens

Ingredients:

.

.1 teaspoon smoked paprika
.1 tablespoon cider vinegar
.½ teaspoon hot sauce
.1/8 teaspoon kosher salt
.1/8 teaspoon freshly ground black pepper
1 tablespoon vegetable oil
.1 yellow onion, diced
.1 collard greens bunch, roughly chopped
.2 cups vegetable broth

Directions:

1. Using the pressure cooker in the sauté or brown mode, proceed to heat the vegetable oil until it reaches its shimmering point. Blend the onion thoroughly, ensuring frequent stirring, until it is softened and translucent, approximately for a duration of 5 minutes. Incorporate the collard greens, vegetable stock, and paprika.

2. Secure the lid tightly and adjust the timer to a duration of 20 minutes on a high setting. When the clock is not in use, it is advisable to let it discharge for approximately ten minutes. After that, proceed to completely remove the cover.

3. Incorporate the vinegar, hot sauce, salt, and pepper. Serve hot.

4. To prepare the collard greens, thoroughly rinse the leaves by immersing them in a sink filled with cold water. Fold the leaves in half along the stem and employ a chef's knife to remove the most rigid portion of the stem. Next, carefully layer several leaves together, rolling them into a cylindrical

shape, and swiftly cut them into broad strips. If desired, you may also choose to further cut the strips.

What Shouldn't You Eat?

The prevailing consensus among clinical experts is that infections primarily arise due to our dietary practices. In addition to the immediate ramifications such as cardiovascular ailments and weight-related concerns, there are also myriad underlying issues that arise from consumption of inappropriate food choices. Taking all factors into account, it is evident from the accumulated data that the prevalence of obesity has experienced a significant surge, rising from 5% to 40% over the course of the past forty years.

Moreover, esteemed professionals have indicated that approximately 60% of the American population is afflicted with chronic ailments, encompassing conditions such as cancer, cardiovascular disorders, clinical depression, as well as Alzheimer's and dementia.

Clinical professionals also propose that diabetes mellitus, another form of chronic illness, is significantly affecting individuals worldwide. There are two types of diabetes - one is part of a category of illnesses known as "autoimmune diseases"; this condition is intractable and cannot be overcome.

Although the initial type is quite traditional, it is the second one that warrants the greatest concern. The second type of diabetes is not an autoimmune disorder; rather, it arises due to excessive sugar consumption, which overwhelms the body's capacity to regulate sugar levels adequately. Presently, a substantial majority of the population experiences Type-2 diabetes, or more commonly known as pre-diabetes. All of these challenges further impact the astuteness and also the political situation of the nation. For example, a significant number of Americans are affected by Type-2 diabetes, and approximately 33% of the funding allocated by Medicare is dedicated to managing diabetic conditions.

This represents a significant amount of funds being allocated towards a critical illness related to the consumption of food. Approximately 70% of aspirants seeking to perpetrate aggression are rejected primarily due to the presence of health conditions such as obesity. A significant number of children within the American context develop by consuming excessively processed and excessively sugary foods, resulting in their becoming overweight and facing significant health complications. This is the rationale for their dismissal from the military.

The innovative food system is exerting an impact on a global scale. There exists a significant abundance of unstimulating culinary options that are improperly managed; moreover, these choices significantly contribute to a substantial portion of our daily nourishment.

In the instance of prebiotic food options, notwithstanding the presumption of having minute digestive tract

Given the presence of an overabundance of bacteria in these food items, it is strongly urged by healthcare professionals to incorporate them into one's diet gradually. While the conventional immune system provides a standardized solution, the adaptable immune system will undoubtedly provide individualized responses to various types of antigens. A paleolithic diet can also aid in strengthening the immune system by reducing the incidence of antigenic challenges such as influenza and common colds.

The existing food system is exerting a significant impact on a global scale. There exist numerous unstimulating food sources that are inadequately processed; these also comprise the majority of our dietary regimen.

Milk

When examining a pegan diet regimen, it presents the notion of considering two distinct dietary approaches - one adhering to the principles of the paleo diet, while the other adheres to the principles of a vegetarian diet. In relation to a vegetarian dietary regimen, dairy products are not endorsed. This is the clarification that milk products exhibit insufficiency in meeting the dietary requirements of a sound vegan regimen. However, many individuals remain perplexed as to the reasons behind advocating for the avoidance of milk. If milk is excluded from a person's diet, despite its proven benefits in promoting strong and healthy bones, why is it still being endorsed? According to individuals with expertise in driving, it is not based on any logical foundation. Undoubtedly, the purported advantages have likewise proven to be unfounded. There exist authentic and perilous hazards such as procedural complications, dermatitis, hormonal imbalances, autoimmune disorders, allergies, as well as malignancies. Myth: Beneficial for skeletal health.

Throughout our adolescence, we have consistently been taught that dairy products constitute the most superior sources of calcium. Consuming such products, renowned for promoting the development of robust bones and reducing the likelihood of fractures, has become an integral component of ensuring our overall health and wellbeing. Clinical specialists concur on the need for diversity. It has been discovered that countries with high milk consumption exhibit a parallel trend with regard to their crack prices, as demonstrated by Sweden. Interestingly, nations with lower milk consumption, such as Indonesia and China, are shown to have correspondingly lower crack prices. A recent study has revealed that the consumption of a daily glass of milk among adults has been associated with a 9% increase in the likelihood of experiencing bone fractures.

By proactively avoiding the consumption of milk, you may find yourself contemplating alternative means to adequately fulfill your calcium and Vitamin D requirements. To begin with, milk has been fortified with Vitamin D, as it is not naturally occurring. In terms of the most advantageous sources of Vitamin D, one could opt for options such as exposure to natural sunlight, consumption of herring, and inclusion of porcini mushrooms in their diet. However, it is also possible to acquire

Calcium can be obtained from sources such as canned salmon, chia seeds, sardines, sesame seeds, tofu, and various leafy greens including arugula, collards, and kale.

What dairy products are you able to consume?

There is a limited selection of dairy products that you may occasionally consume. One can partake in consuming dairy products derived from sheep and goats (or even buffalo), which contain a higher content of A2 casein protein and exhibit lower levels of inflammation. On the other hand, it should be noted that dairy products derived from cows contain significant quantities of A1 casein, a protein known to be associated with the development of dermatitis, acne, allergic reactions, and inflammation. During the interim period, it is worth noting that A2 casein encompasses a potent naturally occurring detoxifying agent, as well as an antioxidant and anti-inflammatory substance called glutathione. Irrespective of your personal preference for cow dairy, it is strongly recommended that you opt for cow products that are of the full-fat variety, derived from grass-fed cows, and produced through regenerative-raised practices.

Both Coffee and Alcohol

Excessive intake of alcoholic beverages and excessive consumption of coffee can induce alterations in one's mood, sleep pattern, and hormonal balance. H2O is the primary beverage that your body requires.

The human body is primarily constituted of water. Inadequate water consumption has the potential to induce a range of illnesses. Irrespective of the desire to infuse water with flavor, one can opt to enhance its taste by adding cucumber or lime, or alternatively, by preparing chilled herbal teas. While it is permissible to consume alcoholic sparkling water on a pegan diet plan, it is highly recommended to prioritize the intake of plain water.

On the contrary, it is also possible to dissolve electrolytes in water; electrolytes refer to minerals that enable the replenishment of bodily mass and nerve function. In doing so, electrolytes aid in waste elimination, cell regeneration, pH balancing, and overall hydration of the body. After engaging in physical exercise, it is advisable to replenish your body with electrolytes in water, as they effectively hydrate your body and replenish the minerals that are lost during the exertion.

Coffee

Coffee is widely regarded as one of the prime sources of antioxidants, which can be utilized to assess the diminished intake of antioxidants consumed in contemporary society. It is evident that espresso possesses a number of advantages - scientific research has unequivocally demonstrated that espresso can effectively reduce the likelihood of various health conditions such as Parkinson's disease, dementia, as well as cardiovascular ailments.

Nonetheless, espresso does not offer assistance to every individual. Generally speaking, espresso has the capacity to increase insulin production, particularly among individuals diagnosed with Type-2 diabetes mellitus. Furthermore, it has the potential to contribute to hormonal damage by elevating stress hormones such as cortisol.

If you are facing heart palpitations, insomnia, or other manifestations of heightened energy, it would be advisable to examine your habitual consumption of coffee. It is advisable to abstain from alcohol consumption intermittently throughout the year. Many of us have become excessively dependent on irrefutable amounts of caffeine to the extent that we cannot initiate our day without a cup of coffee. It has been evidenced that one can experience a commonplace day, even in the absence of the beverage.

Instead of espresso, you could engage in experimenting with several alternative beverages. Tea is an excellent choice due to its abundant presence of potent phenolic compounds that provide protection to our cardiovascular system and possess anti-carcinogenic properties. Similarly, in the event that one cannot live without espresso, it is advised to consume it unflavored and without any additional sweeteners. Alcohol

Numerous individuals assert that opting for a glass of red wine is the most favorable option in comparison to other alcoholic beverages, citing its inclusion of resveratrol. This substance is also present in various supplements and dietary sources.

It has been determined that alcohol significantly impacts females more than males; extensive research has substantiated that women who consume higher quantities of alcohol are markedly more susceptible to developing breast cancer. Additionally, it adversely affects the nutrients present within your body, as well as your cognitive functions, gastric health, and hepatic function. Contrary to conventional belief, alcohol does not facilitate the process of falling asleep; in fact, it can prolong the time it takes to doze off. Additionally, the consumption of alcohol leads to a sustained elevation in heart rate throughout the night.

Consequently, it is imperative to abstain from consuming alcohol. In the event that you are unable to do so, it is advisable to manage alcohol in a manner similar to sugar - the occasional sip is acceptable. It will undoubtedly pose a risk if one consumes on a daily basis. Cease any consumption of alcohol if you do not experience a positive state of well-being subsequent to its consumption. There is no shame in allowing individuals to understand that you do not partake in the consumption of alcohol or that you have indeed abstained. Irrespective of the presence of peer pressure, ascertain to firmly decline and convey to them that you are presently enjoying yourself, even in the absence of alcohol consumption.

White Flour

In this context, our focus is not on beetroot sugar, but rather on the concept of an organic alternative sweetener. Similar to high-fructose corn syrup, beet sugar is genetically modified; however, it is worth noting that raw sweetener does not undergo such modification.

However, it is still acknowledged that both substances have comparable effects on increasing the body's insulin levels, resulting in weight gain (specifically abdominal fat), fatty liver, and prediabetic symptoms such as insulin resistance, diabetes, elevated cholesterol, and so forth.

There is an absence of sanitizing agents in white sugar; moreover, white flour contains bleaching agents. The process by which the sugars in sugar cane are handled involves the extraction of nutrients and minerals, known as molasses, leaving behind only the white sugar. If you do not possess them, the body shall assuredly resort to drawing upon the contents of the books to dissolve the sugar.

Similarly, when the quality of the flour is enhanced, it enables the absorption of vital minerals and nutrients by the body. Given the fact that numerous flour products are fortified, they will undeniably contain artificial nutrients and iron. However, it is important to note that this form of iron does not align with the specific dietary requirements of the human body. These dietary supplements have the potential to pose obstructions to the body, particularly if one has an aversion to iron.

It is profoundly remarkable how the human body expels iron, as the natural tendency is for our bodies to accumulate it rather than eliminate it. Consequently, if you are consuming food containing excess iron from an unreliable source, it can lead to a multitude of potential issues. Likewise, white flour utilizes a combination of conditioners to guarantee ease of transforming the batter into dough and loaves of bread. The flour also incorporates a relaxation agent known as benzoyl peroxide, which can interact with certain essential proteins found in wheat, such as gluten. This interaction produces alloxan, a compound known to induce the destruction of insulin-producing cells in the pancreas. Ultimately, this process leads to the development of Type-1 diabetic conditions in rodents, notably hamsters and mice.

Similarly, flour harbors a hazardous component known as potassium bromate, which is forbidden in Europe, Brazil, China, and Canada. Research has concluded that potassium bromate elicits the formation of malignant cancer cells in animal subjects. When preparing breads, croissants, or biscuits, the additive is employed in white flour to achieve an optimum texture in the dough. In conclusion, white flour also contains gluten, which poses a significant challenge for a considerable portion of the global population. Consuming gluten can activate an immune system reaction, thereby leading to inflammation within your gastrointestinal system.

The latest situation presents a greater magnitude of concerns compared to the previous instance when you juxtapose the color white.

Refined sugar and bleached wheat flour.

Eliminating Sugar Cravings

Numerous individuals struggle with effectively eliminating sugar cravings in a natural manner. There are individuals who struggle to adhere to dietary regimen due to their initial cravings for sugar.

There will inevitably come a time when the craving for sugar, especially carbohydrates such as desserts, grains, bread, and pasta, will overpower you. If you desire to curb your sugar cravings, there are four fundamental steps that you can undertake. These comprise of:

1. Diet plan.

Your dietary plan is the starting point for everything. The primary objective you genuinely aim to achieve is incorporating dietary sources that have the ability to regulate both your blood sugar levels and insulin. Currently, insulin is a naturally occurring substance within the human body that functions in close conjunction with the pancreas. to drop glucose levels. The primary challenge faced by individuals with diabetes is the impaired ability to absorb glucose or the malfunctioning of their insulin receptor sites; additionally, insufficient insulin production within their body may also occur.

To effectively combat your sugar cravings, it is imperative to diligently regulate your insulin levels in order to maintain a stable glucose balance. In order to achieve this, it is highly recommended to incorporate three essential components into your dietary regimen - namely, wholesome and balanced fats, nutritious proteins, and an adequate amount of dietary fiber. These three supplements will undeniably aid in regulating one's glucose levels and effectively curb sugar cravings. You will indeed experience an extended duration of sensation.

Several noteworthy attributes of proteins include organically sourced grass-fed beef, wild game such as turkey and hen, and free-range eggs. You also have the option to select dairy products that are aged. These food sources will enable you to obtain high-quality and, moreover, naturally derived proteins that are beneficial for your health. Consuming additional sound protein will effectively mitigate the desire for sugary foods.

The additional aspect you need is comprised of nutritious and well-balanced fats. You may consider options such as nuts and seeds; noteworthy choices include flax seeds and cultivated chia seeds. Additional remarkable alternatives for incorporating nutritional soundness and adjusted fats consist of clarified butter (ghee), avocados, coconut oil, and almonds. Healthy fats play a crucial role in regulating blood sugar levels.

Fiber is also essential in regulating blood glucose levels. The most

Prominent sources of dietary fiber are derived from various seeds, berries, vegetables, and nuts.

2. Eliminating sugar and grains from your dietary regimen. If you are looking to reduce sugar cravings, it is advisable to eliminate sugars and grains from your diet. This is a significant perpetuating cycle whose effect is that the greater amount of sugar consumed, the higher

the body's demand for it becomes. The initial couple of days following the cessation of sugar consumption will undoubtedly present the greatest challenges.

It is advised by experts to gradually eliminate sugar from your dietary regimen and explore nutritious alternatives that can help satisfy cravings for sweetness. You may incorporate natural stevia powder or leaves into your dietary regimen, as these constituents are likely to assist in addressing any desire for sweetness that you may experience.

Furthermore, you have the option of selecting a protein powder that is rich in taste. Ultimately, it is necessary to eliminate sugar, grains, and starches from your system. 3. Utilizing superior dietary supplements for the purpose of regulating blood glucose levels.

Chromium is a highly beneficial dietary supplement for individuals with diabetes. However, the consumption of 200-micrograms of chromium three times daily can aid in stabilizing blood sugar levels. One can access online retailers to search for premium chromium supplements, which may be ingested alongside meals as a means of regulating blood glucose levels and curbing sugar cravings.

Additionally, you may want to contemplate the incorporation of Vitamin B. The consumption of B-complex vitamins may help overcome sugar cravings, particularly Vitamins B6 and B12. Additionally, there are also probiotic supplements available. These supplements have the potential to mitigate sugar cravings by eliminating yeast from the body. Yeast and detrimental microorganisms derive sustenance from sugar. The supplement will undeniably aid in maintaining a harmonious yeast equilibrium within the body.

These three varieties of dietary supplements will effectively reduce cravings for sugar.

4. Engage in the most effective forms of exercise.

Engaging in an extensive regimen of cardiovascular exercises can lead to an increase in one's propensity for sugary food cravings. Conversely, engaging in isometric or weight-training exercises such as Pilates, yoga, and similar activities can effectively regulate blood sugar levels without inducing carbohydrate cravings. It is advisable to refrain from engaging in long-distance cardiovascular activities such as running, as they can trigger heightened sugar cravings in the body.

Initiating The Foundation Of Adhering To The Pegan Diet

I would like to extend my congratulations to those embarking on their journey with the Pegan Diet, as it reflects a commendable decision to prioritize the improvement and cultivation of their nutritional and overall well-being. I sincerely hope that your decision to embrace the Pegan diet stems not from external influences such as peer pressure, but rather from your genuine commitment to enhance your well-being. Furthermore, I express my desire for our enduring companionship in the foreseeable future. If I may caution you, however, it must be emphasized that embarking on this journey will not be without its challenges. Nevertheless, by diligently adhering to these compelling measures designed to guarantee your steadfast adherence to the Pegan diet, the path ahead will be considerably smoother. Based on the success stories of numerous individuals, I have a strong belief that by demonstrating your unwavering commitment, exercising patience, and showcasing unwavering dedication, you will be well on your way to realizing your aspirations of leading a health-conducive lifestyle and preserving the environment.

When considering dietary patterns and nutritional requirements, there does not exist an ideal diet that suits every individual. This phenomenon may stem from the inherent variations in individual body metabolism and the distinct impact of different foods on bodily functions. In addition, it is important to consider the existence of potential health conditions and allergies, as these factors can significantly influence the impact of dietary regulations and guidelines on a person. In essence, when contemplating the adoption of any diet, it is essential to consider the two main inquiries that determine its suitability for you.

The questions are:

How is my physical well-being?

Which signs and symptoms, if any, am I currently manifesting that may indicate nutrient deficiency and imbalance? These asymmetries may manifest as bloating, constipation, hormonal disruptions, alterations in digestion, fragility of nails or hair, or a catalyst to any latent illness.

Properly addressing these questions can assist in determining the crucial nutrients that may have been lacking in your previous dietary regimen and identifying the nutrients that will be necessary in the prospective Pegan diet you are contemplating.

When adhering to a Pegan Meal Plan, it is important to take the following into consideration:

• Construct your meals with a focus on vegetables.

• Incorporate approximately 1-2 portions of nutrient-rich fats

• Incorporate a generous amount of protein into the majority, if not all, of your meals. Protein should ideally be served in a portion that is equivalent to a condiment.

• Endeavor to limit the consumption of foods that have the potential to provoke inflammation. Inflammatory foods are known to induce sensations of bloating, excessive gas, or constipation. These food items are primarily undergoing processing and packaging.

Now, let us examine the composition of a typical meal that adheres to the principles of the Pegan Diet, as well as the specific food items that you will likely need to incorporate into your dietary regimen.

In the context of carbohydrates, it is recommended that your meal composition should consist of approximately fifty percent (one-third) to a maximum of sixty-six percent (two-thirds) of your plate. The recommended carbohydrate-rich foods to incorporate into your diet consist of broccoli, cauliflower, Brussels sprouts, different varieties of squash, green beans, asparagus, carrots, beets, plantains, sweet potatoes, and a selection of fresh organic fruits. In the event that you wish to incorporate grains and legumes, it is recommended to utilize soaked and sprouted beans.

Proteins constitute a significant portion of the Pegan diet, however, they should be consumed in moderation rather than in large quantities at once. Alternatively, it is recommended to incorporate proteins evenly across all meals throughout the day. Given this scenario, it is recommended that the proportion of protein in your meals should constitute approximately a quarter (1/4) or one-third (⅓) of your plate. In your Pegan diet meal plans, protein sources should consist of organically sourced, pasture-raised, and plant-fed options. This includes locally sourced chicken, wild-caught fish, beef derived from organic animals, eggs, broths, and other organic meat varieties.

Fats ought to be included in the meals adhering to the principles of the Pegan diet. One should only partake in the intake of healthy fats, and the quantity thereof should be kept to a minimum. Each meal ought to consist of approximately twenty-five to thirty-three percent of fat content. Nutritious dietary fats can be sourced from ingredients such as coconut butter, avocado oil, dairy products derived from grass-fed livestock, avocados, coconuts, yogurt, as well as an array of nuts and seeds.

Adhering to fats that have undergone minimal processing is an additional method by which the Pegan diet meal plan can be adopted and adhered to. While it is true that there is a proliferation of processed fats and other processed foods in contemporary society, it is imperative to acknowledge that despite their ubiquity, there is also a wide availability of healthy fats. Nevertheless, it is imperative that these be minimized to the utmost degree possible.

Animal protein should be included in the average Pegan meal, serving as a complete source of protein, for approximately two meals per day. While it can be challenging for individuals to accept that animal-derived protein should be included in their diet, it is crucial to recognize that animal-sourced proteins are the sole form of food that contains complete protein.

As the Pegan Diet incorporates elements from both the Paleo diet and the Vegan diet, it transcends the specific components and guidelines of each individual diet. Instead, it adopts a comprehensive perspective to assess which dietary aspects bear greater influence on human health and physiology. The Pegan diet also promotes the optimal utilization of the Paleo and Vegan diets for the purpose of attaining the utmost level of well-being.

What Advantages Does The Pegan Diet Offer?

The pegan diet gives significant importance to consuming fruits and vegetables that are rich in nutrients, resulting in numerous positive effects on one's health. Fruits and vegetables possess substantial amounts of dietary fiber, as well as essential vitamins, minerals, and antioxidants, all of which play key roles in promoting disease prevention. Omega-3 fatty acids derived from seafood, legumes, and nuts have the potential to enhance cardiovascular health, while adhering to the pegan diet's principle of consuming whole, unrefined food is indeed effective in reducing inflammation.

Consumables

The pegan diet emphasizes the consumption of wholesome grains, which are either minimally processed or completely unprocessed prior to being served.

Incorporate a diverse selection of botanical specimens into one's diet.

The primary food categories in the pegan diet consist of vegetables and fruits, which should comprise approximately 75% of your total dietary intake.

In order to mitigate the response of elevated blood sugar levels, it is advisable to give preference to fruits and vegetables with a low glycemic index, including berries and non-starchy vegetables.

Individuals who have effectively upheld optimal blood sugar levels prior to commencing the dietary regimen may be allowed limited portions of starchy vegetables and fruits with higher sugar content.

Choose Protein That Has Been Sourced from Verified Safe Sources.

If the primary emphasis of the pegan diet lies in plant-based nutrition, it is additionally advisable to ensure adequate intake of protein derived from animal sources.

Please be mindful that given that vegetables and meat make up 75% of the overall diet, animal-based proteins constitute less than one-quarter of the dietary composition. Consequently, your meat consumption will be significantly lower compared to a conventional paleo regimen, yet still considerably higher compared to a vegan dietary approach.

The pegan diet enforces a strict restriction on the consumption of conventionally farmed meats and eggs. In addition to that, it places particular focus on the rearing of grass-fed, pasture-raised cattle, pork, chickens, and whole eggs.

Moreover, it encourages the intake of fish, specifically those that are low in mercury, such as sardines and wild salmon.

Incorporate Fats with Minimal Refinement into Your Diet.

Within this dietary plan, individuals are encouraged to incorporate a diverse range of sources that offer nourishing fats, which can include the following options:

Any variety of nuts, with the exception of peanuts.

With the exception of refined seed oils, all types of seeds are included.

Furthermore, it is worth noting that cold-pressed oils derived from olives and avocados can also serve as a viable alternative.

Unrefined coconut oil is permissible as cocoa.

Omega-3 fatty acids, particularly those sourced from fish not contaminated with mercury or from algae.

Furthermore, the inclusion of grass-fed, pasture-raised meats and whole eggs serves to enhance the fat content within the pegan diet.

The consumption of certain varieties of whole grains and legumes is permissible.

Whilst most grains and legumes are forbidden on the pegan diet as they have the potential to impact blood sugar levels, certain gluten-free whole grains and legumes are permissible to be consumed in limited quantities.

It is recommended that the intake of grains per meal be limited to a maximum of 1/2 cup (125 grams), while the consumption of legumes should not exceed 1 cup (75 grams) per day.

You are required to ingest the following types of grains and legumes:

The assortment comprises black rice, quinoa, amaranth, millet, teff, and oats.

Lentils, chickpeas, black beans, and pinto beans are included.

Nonetheless, individuals who are afflicted with diabetes or any other condition resulting in impaired blood sugar control should exercise even further restraint when consuming these particular foods.

05. Vegan Paleo Pancakes

Vegan Paleo Pancakes exhibit a delicate texture on the interior and achieve a subtly light and fluffy consistency on the exterior. An exquisite pancake option that caters to individuals adhering to an egg- and grain-free dietary regimen. To enhance the taste even more, you can gracefully pour a generous amount of Roasted Strawberry Vanilla Bean Sauce.

List of required ingredients:" "Required ingredients:" "Essential ingredients:"

"Necessary ingredients: " "Requisite ingredients:

One cup of almond flour

Three-fourth cup of tapioca flour

One tablespoon of baking soda.

Ingredients required: A quarter teaspoon of sea salt.

Two-thirds of a cup of unsweetened almond milk.

Two tablespoons of apple cider-derived vinegar

One tablespoon of maple syrup

1 tablespoon of coconut oil, that has been melted

1 teaspoon of pure vanilla extract.

Directions

01. Incorporate all of the ingredients together in a mixer. Operate the blender

for a brief duration, subsequently halt, utilize a utensil to remove any residue from the periphery, and resume blending for an additional brief duration. Additionally, it is possible to prepare the batter in a bowl. However, as previously stated, the use of blending techniques aids in achieving a lighter texture for these pancakes that do not contain eggs.

02. If deemed necessary, incorporate extra liquid or flour in small increments (1/2 tablespoon). Gradually, add milk (in small increments) while stirring the batter, until it reaches the desired consistency akin to pancake batter.

03. Transfer the batter into a skillet that has been greased, ensuring to pour approximately 1/4 cup of batter per pancake, and cook over medium to medium-high heat.

04. Turn the pancakes once they start to form bubbles, as failure to do so

promptly may result in the spatula becoming easily submerged beneath the pancake. Proceed with the cooking process until both sides acquire a desirable golden brown hue.

05. Kindly ensure that the pancakes are given ample time to cool down before being served.

Additional options for toppings include Roasted Strawberry Vanilla Bean Sauce and almond butter, which may be selected as accompaniments.

What Are The Primary Advantages Of Adhering To The Pegan Diet?

Upon thorough analysis of the attributes, origins, and underlying principles of the Pegan diet, it is now appropriate to elucidate the myriad advantages that can be derived from adopting this dietary approach. In the initial section, our focus shall primarily be on the overarching advantages conferred by this dietary regimen, whereas in the subsequent segment, we will delve into the precise benefits it offers for specific ailments.

Nevertheless, the overall advantages of adhering to this dietary regimen include:

• Initially, it serves as a nutritious dietary regimen. As previously mentioned, the Pegan diet embodies a well-rounded and nutritious dietary approach that adequately fulfills all dietary requirements. Despite its consistent preference for proteins and fats over carbohydrates, this regimen offers essential vitamins and minerals through the inclusion of vegetables, which are not typically found in alternative low-carbohydrate diets. This diet does not eliminate any vital component necessary for the body's function. Conversely, it offers a comprehensive array of essential nutrients that are necessary for optimal energy and functionality.

• This dietary regimen is intended to promote overall health and well-being, encompassing benefits for various aspects of our body, including enhancements to the functioning of the digestive system, liver, and mental state. Not only will you observe a substantial enhancement in your gastrointestinal well-being and improved skin complexion, but you will also experience significant advancements in cognitive functionality. One will come to the realization that they exhibit heightened levels of concentration and performance when engaging in tasks demanding greater mental exertion, such as undertaking a job that necessitates cognitive effort. Furthermore, due to the heightened consumption of fruits and vegetables, there has been a notable surge in dietary fiber intake, leading to advantageous outcomes for cardiovascular wellness and disease prevention, particularly pertaining to the colon.

• The dietary regimen is intended for extended use: In connection with the aforementioned, as a well-balanced diet that exerts a positive impact on overall well-being, it has the potential to serve as a protocol (unlike other low carbohydrate diets such as Keto, which must be adhered to only briefly to prevent bodily harm) that can be sustained over a prolonged duration. The designation of Pegan as the "365 diet" is in recognition of its suitability for year-round adherence. This is due to the fact that, as previously observed, it adheres to an annual formula comprising a harmonious combination of proteins, vegetables, beneficial fats, and dietary fibers, progressively mitigating the imbalance that tilts towards carbohydrates.

• It caters to a wide range of individuals. After rigorous examination and analysis, it has been found that the Pegan diet possesses the ability to meet a diverse range of requirements, rendering it suitable for universal adoption.

It is a dietary regimen characterized by a structured framework, which is amenable to customization. Additionally, the Pegan diet emphasizes the utilization of a efficient formula for tailoring meals, known as the 5-4-3-2-1 approach. This numerical sequence serves as a guide for aligning the intake of proteins, carbohydrates, vegetables, fats, and fibers, ensuring a well-balanced nutrition.

• It continues to yield immediate outcomes: despite its potential for long-term implementation and adherence, the Pegan diet offers prompt benefits in terms of weight loss and overall health enhancement. It remains a low-carbohydrate protocol designed to facilitate rapid weight loss.

• Enhances metabolic functions: Due to its focus on dietary re-education, this diet certainly influences and enhances your metabolic efficiency. Opting for minimally processed, low-glycaemic foods that are rich in essential nutrients is also effective in rectifying a compromised metabolism. In conjunction with physical exercise, it will prove to be a highly advantageous companion in achieving sustainable outcomes, particularly with regards to our metabolic system.

• Mitigates stress-induced overeating: By effectively regulating blood sugar levels and minimizing sugar intake, this dietary approach facilitates a substantial decrease in reliance on sugary foods. Furthermore, it is widely recognized that this dependency is the primary catalyst for indulging in stress-driven consumption of food.

• This dietary approach not only revolutionizes our eating habits but also transforms our overall way of living: as a regimen focused on food re-education, it enables us to grasp the essence of healthier food choices, thus lending itself to becoming an authentic lifestyle. The principle underlying the Pegan diet involves the exclusion of processed and industrialized foods, along with sugars and starches, in favor of plant-based foods, protein-rich sources, and nutritious fats. Indeed, in actuality, the exclusion of foods derived from animals is not absolute; rather, they can be ingested provided that they originate from certified organic and environmentally-friendly farms. Consequently, it becomes a question of deliberate ingredient selection and personally preparing our own meals. This novel perspective on the nourishment we consume will undeniably exert an influence on our behaviors and way of life.

• The Pegan diet adheres to an environmentally conscious approach as it promotes the conscious selection of locally sourced and organic food options to minimize the use of harmful chemicals, additives, and pesticides. The aforementioned factors also have a diminished effect on the environmental well-being in our vicinity.

The aforementioned benefits encompass all the potential advantages that can be derived from adhering to the Pegan diet. In the forthcoming chapter, we will elucidate and demonstrate all the unique benefits directly relevant to diabetes and cardiovascular ailments, including hypertension.

Benefits of the Pegan diet for individuals with hypotension and diabetes

Thus far, we have comprehended the primary advantages of the Pegan diet in a general context. It has become evident to us that this dietary regimen facilitates weight loss and effectively regulates numerous vital parameters crucial to maintaining bodily health.

By establishing these definitive parameters, we acknowledge our intention to consume dietary choices that promote cholesterol control and diminish the threat of diabetes, cardiovascular ailments, and other conditions that impact gastrointestinal health. From this perspective, the consumption of substantial quantities of dietary fiber, vitamins, and unsaturated fats plays a crucial role in altering these parameters and exerting a preventive effect. Commencing with the regulation of parameters pertaining to bodily welfare, we can delineate the specific advantages relevant to individuals afflicted with diabetes or hypertension.

When discussing the latter, specifically hypertension, we can make reference to the advantages of this dietary regimen with regards to cardiovascular disorders.

This is attributed to the fact that this dietary regimen, devoid of unhealthy fats which contribute to cardiovascular issues, facilitates a reduction in both cholesterol and triglyceride levels within the bloodstream. We are aware that these factors are primarily responsible for this state of discomfort.

Adhering to a diet rich in beneficial fats, specifically omega 3 fatty acids, which constitutes a prominent aspect of this proposition, coupled with the reduction in salt intake, can effectively contribute to the regulation of blood pressure.

Regarding the advantages for individuals afflicted with diabetes, it is noted that this dietary approach aims to minimize the intake of carbohydrates and sugars as a means to maintain stable blood sugar levels. As a diet characterized by a low glycaemic load, it effectively maintains a state of equilibrium in the blood insulin and glucose levels by substantially reducing or eliminating the consumption of refined flours and carbohydrates. Adhering to the Pegan diet has been observed to enhance the manifestations of diabetes, as well as mitigate the symptoms of stress, anxiety, and various ailments linked with blood sugar dysregulation. Recognizing the fact that processed foods yield scant nutritional value, as they consist predominantly of sugars instead of a substantial quantity of nutrients, artificial substances such as dyes, preservatives, and flavor enhancers are also prevalent in these edible products. Moreover, it is crucial to acknowledge that these foods possess addictive properties and serve as a significant catalyst not only for obesity but also for diabetes globally.

In any event, this dietary regimen is advantageous for mitigating the various perils associated with diabetes as well as those pertaining to cardiovascular health and blood pressure.

We are solely discussing measures of containment or preventive intervention for these diseases, as it is widely acknowledged that dietary modifications alone do not suffice as a solution for these issues, particularly for individuals with more severe conditions.

The Pegan diet, although beneficial, is not entirely sufficient on its own. It is imperative that we consistently emphasize the fundamental medical viewpoint and conduct the requisite evaluations, not merely prior to initiating such a dietary regimen, but also before embarking on any other dietary plan.

Furthermore, when it comes to administering medications, it is imperative that you remember to align your dietary habits accordingly.

Having presented all the benefits associated with this dietary regimen in terms of disease prevention and management, we will now proceed to outline the potential adverse effects or contraindications.

Are there any major adverse effects or precautionary considerations associated with the Pegan diet?

We have thoroughly examined all the potential advantages associated with the Pegan diet. Similar to all dietary regimens, including the Pegan diet, potential issues or contraindications may arise.

In this paragraph, we will succinctly enumerate them, as their number is not considerable.

• One of the primary issues pertains to the inflexibility of the dietary regimen. It continues to adhere to a low carbohydrate dietary approach, in which there is a significant decrease in one of the primary macronutrients, namely sugars. This considerable decrease renders this dietary plan excessively inflexible. Notwithstanding the fact that the Pegan diet presents a comparatively more lenient approach than either a vegan or Paleo diet in isolation, it is worth noting that several of the prescribed limitations impose unwarranted restrictions on highly nutritious food items, including a majority of legumes, whole grains, and dairy products. Advocates of the Pegan diet frequently highlight a rise in the levels of inflammation and blood sugar. This dietary adjustment is necessitated by the need to remove these specific foods in response to an extended period of elevated protein consumption. In the larger scheme, our discourse invariably steers towards the notion that, once the objective of attaining the desired weight is accomplished, there is an imperative to subsequently augment the consumption of carbohydrates. The capricious eradication of substantial food categories may also result in insufficiencies of essential nutrients, particularly if appropriate replacements or alternative nutrient-rich foods are not carefully chosen or considered. Hence, possessing a fundamental understanding of nutrition may be necessary in order to adopt the Pegan diet in a secure manner.

• The diet might incur significant costs and may not be easily attainable for everyone. While the notion of adhering to a diet encompassing an abundance of organically grown fruits, vegetables, and ethically raised meats may appear highly favorable in principle, its implementation may prove unattainable for a considerable number of individuals. This is due to the fact that not all individuals may have access to nearby small pastures. Conversely, the absence of markets or supermarkets in close proximity that offer organic produce and vegetables. Furthermore, the financial implications associated with adopting such a diet should not be overlooked.

• Prolonged adherence to this diet may lead to adverse effects: Despite its origins in the combination of the Paleo and vegan diets, and its potential suitability for long-term adherence, there is a possibility that this diet could eventually manifest the inherent challenges often associated with high-protein diets. As previously stated, aside from detrimentally impacting blood sugar levels, it may also have adverse repercussions on the kidneys and liver, as they are burdened with the task of eliminating excessive byproducts resulting from the breakdown of animal proteins, particularly uric acid.

• It may entail a higher level of complexity to adhere to: the matter at hand is not simply following one diet, but rather following two. Furthermore, as a result of the amalgamation of both diets, you may encounter challenges in integrating foods and formulating meals that adhere to the dietary restrictions. Nevertheless, the conspicuous decrease in dietary carbohydrates obtained from grains elicits uncertainty, primarily due to its potential to pose significant challenges in adhering to such a regimen. In order for the dietary regimen to yield favorable results, it is imperative that you dedicate a substantial amount of time towards meal preparation, possess proficiency in culinary practices and meal organization, and have the means to acquire a diverse selection of potentially costly food items. Furthermore, as a result of the limitations imposed on commonly processed food items like cooking oils, it can be challenging to dine out. This has the possibility to result in increased levels of social isolation or heightened stress levels. Nevertheless, in order to address this issue directly, we have developed a cookbook that caters to individuals who are compelled to labor outdoors and possess limited time to engage in cooking endeavors.

With all conceivable constraints duly considered, we conclude our second chapter. In the ensuing chapter, we shall explore the modification of the Pegan diet, taking into consideration diverse circumstances ranging from pregnancy to athletic endeavors.

How Does This Diet Differ From Other Commonly Adopted Dietary Approaches?

The Pegan diet can be viewed as an amalgamation of various dietary approaches. Nevertheless, it remains distinct from each of them. Allow us to examine the distinguishing characteristics of a Pegan diet in comparison to various other prevalent dietary approaches:

Paleo

According to its definition, the paleo diet espouses the notion that optimal bodily function is achieved by adhering to the eating habits of our ancestors. This dietary plan comprised limited quantities of nuts and seeds, wholesome oils, fruits, vegetables, and meat. It disallowed counterfeit substances, dairy products, legumes, tubers, cereals (including corn), and processed edibles. Lean meats are commonly consumed, and there is no cultivation of crops and grains for agricultural purposes. Typically, the diet would primarily consist of grass and other naturally occurring food sources.

However, a Pegan diet amalgamates the finest aspects of both paleo and vegetarian diets. Therefore, you adhere to a diet consisting of moderate portions of solid oils, natural commodities, vegetables, and meats, while consciously avoiding the consumption of added sugars, gluten, and dairy.

A prominent misconception regarding the paleo diet is that its fundamental composition primarily revolves around the consumption of meat. From a practical standpoint, it would have been inconceivable for mountain men to adhere solely to a diet consisting of meat. It is a challenging endeavor to subdue colossal beings, necessitating a substantial investment of time for tracking and pursuing these entities.

Hence, our ancestors also incorporated the consumption of nutrient-rich foods such as nuts, vegetables, fruits, and legumes as a means of supplementation.

Nevertheless, the similarities between a Pegan and a paleo diet end at this juncture. Due to adherence to a paleo diet, achieving physical fitness becomes notably more challenging since the inclusion of gluten-free grains such as rice, corn, and oats still persists, thereby resulting in a significant calorie surplus. When adhering to a Pegan diet, it is advised to limit your intake of gluten to just one serving.

Vegan

The vegan diet and the Pegan diet exhibit considerable similarities, with the primary distinction lying in the fact that a vegan diet strictly adheres to a 100% plant-based approach, whereas a Pegan diet necessitates a minimum of 75% plant-based foods on one's plate. A vegan lifestyle is characterized by the conscious choice to abstain from the consumption and utilization of any products derived from animals, encompassing not only clothing and food, but also other facets of daily life. Therefore, a vegan diet completely excludes animal-derived food products such as dairy, eggs, and meats.

Individuals choose to adopt a vegetarian diet for a myriad of reasons, ranging from concerns about ecological sustainability to ethical considerations.

Additionally, they can also stem from the desire to enhance overall well-being.

Conversely, a Pegan diet closely resembles a vegetarian diet. Instead of consuming plant-based foods as accompaniments, a Pegan diet incorporates animal-based items as the supporting components. The fundamental components of this dietary regimen consist exclusively of vegetarian options.

Furthermore, a Pegan diet also discourages the consumption of dairy products.

Based on the aforementioned information, it can be concluded that a vegan diet bears a striking resemblance to a Pegan diet. Nevertheless, in the context of a vegan diet, you abstain from the consumption of meat, poultry, and fish. Furthermore, vegans adhere to the exclusion of various additional forms of animal-derived substances from their lifestyles and dietary choices, such as honey and eggs. This stance extends to encompass all products that may contain animal by-products, including leather, wool, cosmetics, and similar items. In the context of a Pegan diet, the consumption of animal-based products is permitted; however, it is essential that these meals comprise only a quarter (25%) of your plate, while the remaining three-fourths (75%) should consist of plant-based foods.

Vegetarian

Certain individuals may choose to adopt a plant-based diet and abstain from consuming meat for a variety of reasons. In accordance with its definition, a vegetarian diet encompasses the exclusion of all culinary items derived from animal sources, such as eggs, dairy products, seafood, poultry, and meat.

Similarly, a vegan diet abstains from all animal-derived products, including fish, poultry, and meat. Nevertheless, they are authorized to partake in a limited selection of animal-derived products such as dairy.

When comparing a vegetarian diet to the Pegan diet, there exist numerous parallels. For instance, both types of dietary regimens encompass the inclusion of plant-based foods.

Nevertheless, this is where the resemblances come to a halt. When engaging in a Pegan diet, it is strictly prohibited to consume any dairy products such as margarine, milk, and so forth.

Furthermore, you are also prohibited from consuming grains in their entirety or processed form.

Contrary to the Pegan diet, the consumption of various animal-based products such as meat, eggs, and meat is strictly prohibited. Nevertheless, this also depends on the type of vegan diet you are adhering to. Take, for instance, the flexitarian diet, more formally recognized as the semi-vegetarian diet, which encompasses the consumption of dairy products and eggs. This dietary approach also incorporates small portions of fish, seafood, poultry, and meat. Furthermore, the Pescatarian diet excludes the consumption of poultry and meat, but allows for the consumption of seafood, fish, dairy products, and eggs.

Keto

The emphasis varies between the Pegan diet and the keto diet, despite both being focused on plant-based eating patterns. A ketogenic diet exhibits a strong preference for plant-based food options;

conversely, a Pegan diet shares a similar inclination towards the paleolithic regime. Although there are multiple similarities between the two, there are also distinct variations that should be noted.

The renowned clinical professional, Will Cole, is credited with the creation of the ketogenic diet. He ultimately transitioned to ketogenic diets after witnessing their efficacy among his patients. Although some individuals adhere to a keto diet that involves a significant consumption of animal fats and products, Cole modified the dietary approach to solely rely on fish as the primary source of animal protein.

Certainly, it is indeed possible to adhere to a vegetarian variation of the ketogenic diet since the diet is defined by whether one achieves nutritional ketosis. Based on the hypothesis, the method by which one achieves the ketosis state holds no significance; entering into ketosis is achievable regardless of the quality of food consumed, be it low or high in nutritional value.

Both types of diets aim to regulate glucose levels and reduce inflammation. To a large extent, the two weight management programs disregard the inclusion of vegetables, grains, meat, and dairy. The most notable aspect of these weight management programs is that the restrictions imposed are flexible - neither of the plans is excessive or rigid. Additionally, both types of diets allow occasional consumption of "forbidden" foods, as long as it does not give rise to any complications. In broad terms, both types of diets are generally considered to be reliable choices.

DASH

The DASH diet, also known as Dietary Approaches to Stop Hypertension, is a dietary plan meticulously formulated to effectively address hypertension, obviating the need for any pharmacological intervention. This type of diet is also adhered to for the purpose of preventing other forms

pertaining to medical conditions such as diabetes, stroke, and coronary disease

neoplastic formation and demineralization of bones.

A typical DASH diet consists of nuts, poultry, fish, whole grains, low-fat dairy, fruits, and vegetables, bearing a striking resemblance to a Mediterranean diet. In any event, this dietary regimen imposes limitations on sodium intake, permitting no more than 2,300mg of salt per day. Although this diet does not directly result in weight loss, it is often observed that individuals experience a decrease in weight due to their adoption of healthier choices.

In comparison to the Pegan diet, the two eating regimens share numerous similarities. Natural products, vegetables, and animal-derived products constitute a portion of your meal. However, if you aim to ensure the lean quality of the meat in accordance with the principles of the DASH diet, it is crucial that the eggs, poultry, and meat are sourced from humanely raised animals, are organic, and have been fed with grass-based diets, as advocated by the Pegan diet. Although nuts are included in both weight control plans, the Pegan diet excludes whole grains when compared to the DASH diet.

Moreover, the Pegan diet also discourages the consumption of dairy products, in contrast to the DASH diet that allows for the inclusion of a low-fat diet. The dissimilarities between the two diet types converge on the outcome, whereby individuals adhering to DASH diets frequently experience health complications such as hypertension, which can be mitigated by the consumption of aforementioned food items.

Mediterranean Diet

Upon careful examination, it becomes evident that there are minimal disparities between a Mediterranean diet and a Pegan diet. According to reports, adhering to a Mediterranean dietary pattern provides a multitude of advantages ranging from decreased inflammation and weight reduction to diminished susceptibility to prevalent chronic ailments and conditions.

According to extensive research, it has been ascertained that adhering to a Mediterranean diet, along with refraining from smoking and engaging in daily physical activity, can effectively prevent 90% of Type-2 diabetes cases, 90% of coronary heart diseases, and 7% of strokes. You are advised to adhere to the dietary choices that align with the traditional Mediterranean diet, which is known for its high quality standards.

Upon comparing the Mediterranean diet to a Pegan diet, it becomes apparent that both dietary approaches revolve around prioritizing healthier eating patterns. The two dietary plans emphasize the consumption of a greater quantity of vegetables and fruits. The Mediterranean diet adheres to the principles of the paleo diet by refraining from consuming packaged or processed foods.

The primary distinction between the two diets lies in the quality of animal products, with an emphasis on the consumption of pasture-raised, wild-caught, and organic meat. Additionally, the Pegan diet also eliminates processed foods such as bread and whole wheat products. Dairy products are also excluded in a Pegan dietary regimen.

The Distinctive Attributes Of The Pegan Diet In Contrast To Other Prominent Dietary Approaches

The Pegan diet has emerged as one of the most prominent and progressive dietary patterns in recent times. Here's the way by which it piles facing other as lately mainstream food plans.

Paleo

This dietary regimen revolves around specialized animal products such as meat, fish, and eggs, in addition to fats, vegetables, fruits, nuts, and seeds. The Paleo diet restricts the consumption of grains, dairy products, vegetables, sugar, and processed foods. Due to the fact that pegan is derived from paleo, there are numerous similarities present, albeit with notable distinctions. Specifically, pegan allows for the inclusion of certain grains, legumes, vegetables, and locally-sourced dairy products.

Veggie Lover

The alternative aspect that evoked the configuration of pegan, a plant-based regimen, excludes any form of animal-derived products or substances derived from animals that have the capacity for reproduction. It is predicated upon plant-derived food items, while deliberately abstaining from any products derived from animals. The Pegan diet aims to select ecologically conscious and sustainably sourced foods, much like veganism; however, it allows for the inclusion of meat and other animal products to a limited degree. Both veggie enthusiasts and proponents of the pegan diet emphasize the paramount importance of consuming vegetables and fruits.

Vegan

There exists a category of individuals practicing vegetarianism that carries a lesser degree of strictness compared to the more fervent adherents, often referred to as veggie-sweethearts. While certain individuals allow the consumption of fish and eggs, there are those who only sanction the consumption of dairy. Vegetarian individuals may discover a great compatibility in adhering to pegan dietary guidelines, which involve consuming meat and animal products in modest quantities.

Keto

The ketogenic diet primarily consists of a controlled intake of high-fat foods, limited carbohydrates, and a moderate amount of protein. The ketogenic diet consists of a reduced intake of vegetables and natural foods due to their carbohydrate content, while it emphasizes higher consumption of fats and meats compared to the Pegan diet. Although it is possible to adhere to a paleo-keto diet, it presents more challenges to follow a Pegan diet in conjunction with a ketogenic approach due to the inherent difficulty in composing a plate consisting of 75% vegetables and fruits.

DASH

The DASH diet pertains to Dietary Approaches to Stop Hypertension and is typically employed in cases of elevated cholesterol levels, increased risk of coronary disease, or presence of diabetes. Based on a foundation of reduced sodium levels compared to the standard American diet, this approach incorporates an abundance of vegetables, fruits, whole grains, and low-fat dairy. Consume a recommended allowance of 6 to 8 servings of grains per day. It likewise emphasizes a diet rich in lean meats, poultry, and fish, while restricting the consumption of fats and oils to a consistent serving size of 2. Running and walking exhibit contrasting characteristics on several significant factors. Pegan encourages moderate consumption of grains, whereas DASH emphasizes the inclusion of grains as a key component of a balanced diet. Conducting sodium assessments and promoting the consumption of low-fat dairy is advised by the 'run' dietary approach, whereas the 'pegan' dietary approach disregards the consideration of sodium as a constituent when eliminating food assortments. Pegan significantly compromises the integrity of cow's milk-based dairy products.

Mediterranean Diet

The Mediterranean diet, in addition, prioritizes cardiovascular well-being and encompasses several shared principles with the Pegan diet. Both facilitate the consumption of larger quantities of vegetables, through the utilization of vegetable oil, as well as the consistent ingestion of fish. From that point onward, they exhibit contrasts nonetheless. The Mediterranean diet incorporates the promotion of vegetable oils, reduction of sodium intake, increased emphasis on whole grains, and strict limitation of meat consumption to only a few occasions per month. The Pegan diet primarily focuses on incorporating oils in addition to individuals who primarily consume plant-based foods and are restricted to consuming whole grains. While it is not explicitly stated that meat should be the primary food, the pegan diet emphasizes the consumption of high-quality meat within certain limits. In any event, the

Mediterranean diet significantly reduces meat consumption.

Comprehensive Guidelines for Prudently and Efficiently Diminishing Weight by Adhering to a Pegan Regimen

Whenever embarking on a new dietary regimen, it is prudent to consult with your physician. Before embarking on a dietary transition

Obtain baseline blood tests, focusing particularly on inflammatory indicators, lipids, glucose, and insulin levels, as this will set the foundation for further examination and potential outcomes.

— enables you to monitor your progress in terms of how the diet is aiding you in attaining your objectives and enhancing your overall well-being. The quantity of weight lost on the scale should not be perceived as the sole indicators of good health; indeed, improvements in various health indicators frequently occur before measurable weight reduction takes place.

According to Hyman's statement, this pertains to the process of customizing the system, rather than adhering to a predetermined structural design. Certain aspects of the Pegan diet may not be suitable for individuals with diabetes or other medical conditions. It is at this juncture that engaging with your medical team can prove beneficial and establish the groundwork for you. In due course, your dietary requirements may undergo alteration. Pegan often displays adaptability, presenting a respectable degree of customization that adheres to established guidelines.

Precisely, pegan eating revolves not around hardship or prohibition, but rather around the nourishment and contemplation it entails. Maintaining a significant distance from processed and sugary food sources is of great importance; however, this does not imply that one should experience feelings of deprivation. This book presents a multitude of approaches for preparing wholesome meals, snacks, and even indulgent treats using ingredients that align with the principles of pegan cuisine.

Comprehensive Guidelines for Initiating a Pegan Diet

Commencing adherence to a Pegan diet can be approached through various methodologies. This book provides more than 125 patterns to initiate your journey, including a comprehensive meal plan spanning a month of dining. If you are truly determined to proceed, begin by following the dinner itinerary. However, you can also utilize the strategies outlined in this book to become familiar with the Pegan diet over a period of several weeks or even a month in order to fully integrate this improved approach to eating. The plans encompass a user-friendly format that facilitates comprehension. Nevertheless, they are delectable and do not cause any lingering aftertaste commonly associated with "restrictive dietary fare" in the slightest. Pegan is a routine that one consistently adheres to. Alternatively, you may consider implementing an 80/20 system, which proposes adhering to a pegan diet during weekdays and allowing yourself dietary freedom on weekends. The benefits of adopting a pegan diet may not be immediately evident through occasional adherence, but as one increasingly incorporates this approach into their meals, the rewards will become more pronounced.

If embarking on a month-long meal plan appears to be excessively overwhelming, consider incorporating one pegan day into your weekly routine and gradually progress towards incorporating this approach for all seven days. As you familiarize yourself with the dietary guidelines and attain a state of normalcy, the cognitive effort required will diminish, affording you the option to seamlessly incorporate it into your daily routine. Organizing a positive gathering of individuals to enhance the dining experience can also contribute to increased success rates and, consequently, profound satisfaction.

If your partner or relatives do not adhere to the Pegan diet, consider seeking a companion to accompany you. You will mutually share and discuss meals, exchanging suggestions on food preparation and recipe choices, thereby motivating each other to persevere in this endeavor.

The Pegan diet is considered nutritionally sound and suitable for individuals of all demographics, including pregnant and lactating women, as it does not rely on strict calorie restrictions. While advocating for individual promotion can be regarded as unethical, Pegan maintains its legitimacy by virtue of its non-participation.

The approach does not stipulate any specific thresholds and prioritizes substantial quantities of genuine, unprocessed foods with minimal manipulation.

Can The Pegan Diet Be Considered A Nourishing Option For Individuals?

In comparison to the dietary recommendations stipulated by the federal guidelines for a well-balanced eating plan, the pegan diet exhibits an imbalance as it imposes restrictions on the consumption of grains, legumes, and dairy products. The 2020-2025 USDA Dietary Guidelines for Americans recommend the consumption of a diverse range of nutrient-rich foods such as whole fruits and vegetables, legumes, whole grains, lean sources of protein, low-fat dairy products, and healthy fats in order to achieve a balanced diet.

Considering that a pagan diet does not impose any restrictions on daily food intake, it does not inherently contradict the recommendations provided by the USDA for daily calorie consumption, macro- and micronutrient intake. With meticulous strategic consideration, it should be possible for you to fulfill these requirements while adhering to the diet's list of authorized food items.

If one is striving to achieve weight loss, it is beneficial to ascertain one's daily caloric needs to effectively remain aligned with one's objectives. This calculator has the ability to offer an estimation in the event you have a desire to determine calorie content.

The United States Department of Agriculture (USDA) advises the incorporation of dairy, grains, and legumes into a well-rounded and nutritious diet. If you opt for a pagan diet, it may be necessary to exert deliberate effort in meal planning for a diverse range of options, while also ensuring adequate intake of essential nutrients such as calcium, iron, B vitamins, and vitamin D.

HEALTH BENEFITS

Dr. Hyman posits that both plant-based and paleo diets yield comparable health advantages. Indeed, scientific research demonstrates that plant-based diets have the potential to effectively treat and prevent various chronic illnesses, as well as facilitate weight loss. Additionally, paleo diets have shown associations with weight reduction and the management of chronic conditions. However, further investigation is required to ascertain the long-term impacts on health.

Nevertheless, there is no empirical evidence to suggest that the amalgamation of these two regimens and the imposition of limitations on specific food groups can result in more favorable health outcomes than adhering to a properly balanced diet. Although dairy products are often criticized for their high saturated fat content, a comprehensive study conducted in 2016 demonstrated that dairy fat did not display any association with the risk of developing cardiovascular disease.

HEALTH RISKS

Although the pegan diet is a relatively new eating pattern and no known health risks have been associated with it, it is important to note that the exclusion of dairy and whole grains in this diet may result in potential nutrient deficiencies. Cow's milk is rich in essential nutrients such as calcium, protein, potassium, and vitamin D, all of which are vital for overall well-being.

Furthermore, whole grains serve as an excellent source of fiber and vital nutrients. A seminal study conducted in 2016 substantiated the notion that consumption of whole grains reduces the likelihood of developing cardiovascular ailments, cancer, and overall mortality rates. Furthermore, supplementary investigations indicate that inadequate consumption of these nutrients can result in insufficiencies of thiamine, folate, magnesium, calcium, iron, and iodine.

Beans offer a wide array of advantages as well, and are widely recognized as a nutritious food due to their high fiber, protein, and phytonutrient content. Indeed, beans serve as an excellent source of plant-derived protein in numerous vegan dietary regimens. Excluding legumes from a diet that predominantly consists of 75% plant-based foods exposes adherents to the potential risk of inadequate protein, fiber, and essential nutrient intake.

POTENTIAL BENEFITS

The pegan diet may have a beneficial impact on your overall well-being through various means.

The significant focus on the consumption of fruits and vegetables may be considered its most commendable characteristic.

Fruits and vegetables exhibit a significant range of nutritional diversity. They contain a plethora of dietary fiber, essential vitamins, minerals, and botanical compounds renowned for their disease-preventive properties and their ability to mitigate oxidative stress and inflammation.

The pagan diet also places significant emphasis on consuming nutritious, unsaturated fats derived from sources such as fish, nuts, seeds, and various plant-based foods, known to potentially contribute to improved cardiovascular well-being.

In addition, diets that place emphasis on consuming unprocessed foods and have minimal intake of highly processed foods are linked to an enhancement in overall dietary quality.

POTENTIAL DOWNSIDES

Although the pegan diet possesses favorable qualities, it is imperative to contemplate the potential drawbacks it entails.

Unnecessary restrictions

Despite the fact that the pegan diet offers greater flexibility compared to a strictly vegan or paleo diet, several of the suggested limitations needlessly restrict highly nutritious foods, such as legumes, whole grains, and dairy.

Supporters of the pegan diet frequently attribute the exclusion of these foods to higher levels of inflammation and heightened blood sugar as the primary rationales.

Naturally, there are individuals who have allergic reactions to gluten and dairy, resulting in the potential exacerbation of inflammation. Likewise, some individuals face difficulties in regulating their blood sugar levels upon consumption of high-starch foods such as grains or legumes.

In these instances, it may be suitable to decrease or eradicate the consumption of these food items.

Nevertheless, unless you possess particular allergies or intolerances, it is unnecessary to refrain from their consumption.

In addition, the indiscriminate exclusion of substantial food groups may give rise to deficiencies in essential nutrients, unless these nutrients are thoughtfully substituted. Consequently, acquiring a fundamental knowledge of nutrition is advisable in order to safely adopt the pegan diet.

Insufficient accessibility

While the idea of consuming a diet primarily composed of organic fruits, vegetables, and grass-fed, pasture-raised meats may appear highly desirable, it could prove unfeasible for a significant portion of the population.

In order for the dietary regimen to achieve desirable results, a substantial amount of time must be allocated towards the preparation of meals, accompanied by a reasonable level of proficiency in culinary skills and meal planning. Furthermore, access to a diverse range of food items, some of which may carry a higher price tag, is essential.

Furthermore, as a result of the limitations placed on commonly processed food items, such as cooking oils, it may prove challenging to dine out. This could potentially result in heightened social isolation or psychological distress.

The Pegan diet imposes unwarranted restrictions on several essential food groups. It may additionally incur high costs and require significant time investment.

Pizza Made with Mature Yeast Culture

Preparation 20 minutes
cooking 25 minutes
Downtime 24 hours

Portions 4 people
ingredients
Approximately half a kilogram of flour.
A glass containing 300 grams of water.
A quantity of 150 grams of sourdough
that has already been refreshed
and stored at an ambient temperature
for a duration of 4 hours
1 tablespoon of premium quality extra
virgin olive oil.
One teaspoonful of sugar
10 grams of sodium chloride.

Preparation
Combine the mother yeast with the
water, at ambient temperature,
alongside the sugar, in order to dissolve
it. Integrate the flour, 0, oil, and salt,
exerting effort until achieving a cohesive
dough with a smooth consistency. Allow
to rest, covered, at ambient temperature
for a duration of one hour. Subsequently,
proceed to refrigerate the dough for a
duration of 24 hours, ensuring it is

adequately covered. After the allotted time has passed, allow the dough to rest at ambient temperature for a duration of one hour prior to proceeding with the rolling process. You have the option to select between creating a solitary pizza or preparing four individual pizzas. After rolling out the dough, allow it to undergo a further fermentation period of 2 hours. Please ensure to season your pizza(s) according to your personal preference and proceed to cook them in a preheated oven set at 250° for a duration of 25 minutes. The initial twenty can be found in the central region, while the remainder are situated towards the upper section.

Garlic Spinach

Ingredients:

- ¼ teaspoon salt
- ½ lemon, juiced
- ½ tablespoon unsalted butter
- 1 tablespoon garlic powder 2
- cups fresh spinach

Directions:

Choose the Sauté function on the Instant Pot. When the pot reaches a high temperature, incorporate the butter.

2. Incorporate the garlic powder into the mixture while cooking, ensuring it is thoroughly combined until the aroma of

the garlic becomes evident, typically for approximately 30 seconds.

3. Place two small bunches of spinach into the pot simultaneously, ensuring the lid is tightly sealed.

4. Please proceed to shut the strain discharge valve. Choose the "Manual" function and adjust the pot to High Pressure for a duration of 5 minutes.

5. At the completion of the designated cooking period, allow the pot to remain undisturbed for a duration of 10 minutes. Subsequently, release any surplus pressure, incorporate the lemon juice, and season with salt.

Berry Power Smoothie

Ingredients: .

- .1½ cups coconut milk or unsweetened nut milk

- .1/8 teaspoon ground cinnamon (optional)

- ¼ cup frozen blueberries

- .¼ cup frozen strawberries

- .½ cup baby spinach

- .2 tablespoons unsalted almond butter

Directions:

1. Place every one of the fixings into a blender and heartbeat until all around consolidated, around 1 minute.
 2. Pour into a glass and appreciate immediately.

Enchilada With Sweet Potato And Accompanied By A Sauce Of Cilantro And Avocado

Ingredients

- 2 c. peeled and chopped sweet potato
- 15-oz. black beans
- 1 tbsp. freshly squeezed lime juice
- ¼ tsp. sea salt
- ¼ tsp. pepper
- 1 tsp. chili powder
- ½ tsp. ground cumin

- 12 corn tortillas
- ½ tsp. salt
- 3 c. enchilada sauce
- 1 tbsp. olive oil
- 1 chopped red bell-pepper
- 1 chopped red onion
- 2 minced garlic cloves

For Cilantro-Avocado Sauce:

- ½ cup fresh cilantro
- ¼ tsp. sea salt
- ½ tsp. garlic powder
- 1 medium avocado
- 2 tbsps. lime juice

Garnishes:

- Fresh cilantro leaves
- Green sliced onion

Instructions

Prior to use, it is advised to preheat the oven to a temperature of 350 degrees Fahrenheit and apply a light coating of cooking oil.

Simmer the sweet potato in an adequate amount of water within a saucepan. Set the heat to a medium level and allow it to simmer for a duration of 5 minutes. Drain them and reserve.

Place a skillet containing some oil over a medium heat setting, then incorporate the onion and garlic. Proceed to sauté for a duration of 3 minutes, ensuring that the onion achieves a translucent appearance, following which one may proceed to add the desired seasonings.

Incorporate bell pepper, black beans, and pre-cooked sweet potatoes. Increase the temperature to a medium-high setting and proceed to cook for approximately 8 minutes.

Take the skillet off the heat and incorporate ½ cup of enchilada sauce, chili powder, salt, and lime juice.

Ensure a uniform distribution of 1 cup of enchilada sauce over the surface of the greased baking dish. Place the filling evenly into each of the tortillas. Carefully roll the tortillas and position them in the baking dish with the seam facing downwards. Evenly distribute the remaining enchilada sauce onto the tortillas.

Please place the enchiladas in the oven, uncovered, and bake them for approximately 20 minutes, or until the sauce reaches a deep red hue and the enchiladas have heated thoroughly.

During this interim period, prepare a sauce comprised of cilantro and avocado. Utilize the food processor to finely chop the cilantro. Incorporate avocado, salt, lime juice, 2 tablespoons of water, and garlic powder into the mixture and continue processing until a creamy consistency is achieved.

Upon completion of the cooking process for the enchiladas, proceed to individually arrange them, followed by the application of the cilantro-avocado sauce and, if preferred, the addition of green onion and cilantro as a garnish.

Nourishing Chia Pudding For A Satisfying Morning

Ingredients

- 1 teaspoon alcohol-free vanilla extract
- 1 teaspoon maple syrup
- 3 tablespoons chia seeds
- 1 cup of coconut milk

DIRECTIONS

Incorporate all of the specified ingredients into a generously proportioned bowl, employing a delicate stirring motion before securely sealing the container.

Transfer the mixture to your refrigerator and allow it to chill overnight.

The following morning, present the dish alongside your preferred accompaniments.

Banana Fruit Protein Shake

Ingredients:

- 1 cup oat, almond, or cashew milk
- 2 tbsp chia seeds
- 1 scoop of vanilla plant-based protein powder
- Unsweetened coconut shavings
- Papaya seeds
- 1 frozen banana, chopped into smaller sections
- 1 cup frozen strawberries
- 1/2 cup frozen papaya
- 1/2 cup frozen mango chunks

Directions:

Integrate the frozen banana and fifty percent of the milk within a blender. Blend until somewhat combined.

Incorporate frozen fruit into the mixture and thoroughly blend until smooth. If necessary, utilize a spatula to remove any residual ingredients from the sides of the blender to ensure their incorporation. Add the remaining quantity of milk as necessary.

Lastly, incorporate the chia seeds and protein powder by pulsing until they are thoroughly combined.

Transfer the mixture into a tall glass or bowl, then garnish it with coconut shavings and papaya seeds. Enjoy!

Brussels Sprouts With Fava Beans And Turkey In A Tangy Sauce

INGREDIENTS

- 30 ml coconut aminos
- juice of half a lemon
- 12 almonds
- 2 tablespoons apple cider vinegar
- 1 tablespoon honey or agave syrup
- sea salt and pepper
- 500 g Brussels sprouts
- 450 g fresh broad beans
- 250 g turkey breast
- 1 clove of garlic
- coconut oil
- 3 tablespoons sesame seeds

PROCEDURE

Thoroughly cleanse the Brussels sprouts, eliminating any discolored leaves, and proceed to halve them. Heat the oil in a pan, allowing the garlic to achieve a rich golden hue before introducing the sprouts, along with approximately 60 ml of water. Simmer the ingredients over medium heat and cover with a lid until they reach a tender texture and the excess liquid has evaporated. Then, increase the heat to achieve a slight browning.

Slice the turkey breast into small cubes, sear them in a skillet using coconut oil, and generously garnish with lemon juice to achieve a desirable caramelized exterior. Subsequently, immerse freshly harvested broad beans in salted water and allow them to blanch for approximately 8 minutes before incorporating them into the turkey. Proceed by seasoning the mixture with an appropriate amount of salt and pepper.

In a petite bowl, combine honey, vinegar, and prepared aminos. Subsequently, drizzle the mixture over the sprouts, gently stir to infuse the flavors, and proceed to sprinkle the sesame seeds, sliced or diced almonds, salt, pepper, and fava beans with turkey. Agitate gently to enhance the flavors, then proceed to present the dish.

Premium Dark Chocolate Bark Infused With Nutrient-Packed Superfoods

Ingredients

- 2 tablespoons (14 g) chopped pecans
- 2 tablespoons (16 g) pumpkin seeds
- 1 tablespoon (10 g) hemp seeds
- 6 ounces (170 g) 85% or higher dark chocolate
- 1 tablespoon (14 g) coconut oil
- ½ cup (90 g) pomegranate arils, divided

Arrange a compact baking sheet with a piece of parchment paper. Set aside.

Using a bain-marie, heat the chocolate and coconut oil together, continuously stirring until the mixture achieves a smooth and completely melted consistency. Incorporate a quarter cup (45 g) of the pomegranate arils. Transfer the chocolate mixture onto the pre-prepared baking sheet and proceed to evenly distribute it to form a substantial rectangular shape.

Gently distribute the remaining ¼ cup (45g) of pomegranate arils, along with the pecans and seeds, across the surface of the chocolate.

Place in a refrigeration unit for approximately 20 minutes to allow the chocolate to solidify, subsequently divide it into smaller segments.

Store in a chilled environment within a hermetically sealed receptacle for approximately one week, or alternatively, preserve by freezing for a maximum duration of three months. Consume immediately after removing from the freezer in order to prevent melting.

Banana Coconut Cream Pie With Insufficient Crust Base

- ½ cup (113 g) salted butter, melted
- Chocolate Ganache:
- ½ cup (85 g) semisweet
- ½ cup heavy cream

- 1 ½ cups (150 g) graham cracker crumbs, about 11 rectangle graham crackers
- ½ cup (43 g) toasted shredded coconut
- 1 tablespoon brown sugar

Pudding Filling:

- 2 tablespoons butter
- 1 teaspoon vanilla extract
- 1 teaspoon coconut extract
- 2-3 medium bananas, peeled and sliced 1/4-inch thick

- 1 (13-ounce) can of coconut milk
- 1 ½ cups heavy cream
- 3 large egg yolks
- ¾ cup (159 g) granulated sugar
- ⅓ cup cornstarch
- Pinch salt

Topping:

- ¼ teaspoon vanilla extract
- ½ cup (43 g) toasted shredded coconut
- 1 cup heavy whipping cream
- ¼ cup (29 g) powdered sugar

INSTRUCTIONS

Set the oven temperature to 350°Fahrenheit for the crust preheating process. Combine all the ingredients for the crust until they are evenly moistened. Using a 9-inch pie pan, firmly press the mixture into the base and sides. Bake for a duration of 8 to 9 minutes, or until the baked goods acquire a golden brown color. Take the pan out of the oven and place it aside to cool completely.

Utilizing the microwave, proceed to heat the cream until it reaches a boiling point. This process will result in the creation of the ganache. Please position the chocolate chips on the surface. Permit it to rest for a duration of 3-5 minutes, or until the chocolate chips have fully liquefied. Continuously agitate the mixture until it achieves a glossy and velvety consistency. Distribute uniformly across the bottom of the chilled crust. Please keep the pie refrigerated until you are prepared to assemble the remaining portion.

To prepare the pudding, combine the coconut milk, cream (or half-and-half), egg yolks, sugar, cornstarch, and salt in a medium-sized saucepan. Heat the mixture over medium heat, whisking or swirling constantly, until it reaches a gentle simmer. Continue cooking until substantial bubbles emerge on the surface of the concoction, signifying the attainment of desired thickness.

Upon removing the pan from the burner, proceed to promptly incorporate the butter, vanilla, and coconut extracts, subsequently blending all ingredients together using a whisk.

In the event of the pudding's separation or curdling during the preparation process, it is recommended to vigorously whisk it for a brief period of time in order to reintegrate it.

A precision sieve is employed to strain the concoction (although not obligatory, it facilitates the removal of minuscule clumps). The pudding will cool sufficiently in the refrigerator in approximately ninety minutes. To maintain its cool temperature, enclose it within a layer of plastic wrap and store it in the refrigerator.

It is now opportune to consolidate all the elements. In order to ensure comprehensive coverage of the bananas, distribute half of the pudding evenly over them, extending it to the edges in order to prevent any discoloration.

Evenly distribute the remaining pudding over the upper layer, meticulously ensuring its complete coverage of the entire surface. Next, proceed to incorporate an additional layer of banana slices. Evenly distribute the remaining pudding on the surface, ensuring it extends to the outermost edges. Subsequently, placing an additional stratum of sliced bananas on the surface.

Please ensure that the pie is placed in the refrigerator for approximately 1 to 2 hours, or until it has reached a fully cooled state.

The cream, powdered sugar, and vanilla need to be beaten together until they achieve a thick and creamy consistency for the topping (I utilize my blender, although an electric handheld or stand mixer would also suffice).

Additionally, one may choose to garnish the pie with whipped cream and toasted coconut on its surface. At present, the pie is prepared for immediate consumption. It can be served immediately or refrigerated for an additional 1 to 2 hours (prolonged refrigeration may cause the whipped cream to exhibit slight separation and release liquid).